Amoxil

Richard Oliva

Amoxil (amoxicillin): What Is It?

Amoxil (amoxicillin) is a penicillin-type anti-toxin used to treat diseases brought about by microscopic organisms that are B-lactamase negative (B-lactamase positive microbes are generally impervious to Amoxil); These infections typically affect the eye, nose, throat, lungs, skin, and urinary tract. Amoxil comes in the form of a generic drug known as amoxicillin. Amoxil can be made more effective by combining it with other medications, like clavulanic acid (Augmentin).

What are Amoxil (amoxicillin) side effects?

Amoxil's most common side effects include:

nausea, vomiting, diarrhea, stomach pain, itching or discharge from the vagina, a headache, a rash, and a swollen, black, or "hairy" tongue are all symptoms.

Amoxil can also cause serious side effects like:

fever, burning eyes, sore throat, skin pain, seizures, hives, diarrhea that is watery or bloody, red or purple skin rash with blistering and peeling, severe stomach pain, jaundice, and swelling of your face, lips, tongue, or throat are all symptoms of colitis, which is caused by an overgrowth of Clostridium spp. in the intestines.

Amoxicillin dosage Amoxil comes in a variety of forms, including powder for oral suspension and pediatric oral suspension, capsules, tablets, and chewable tablets.

Amoxil can cause serious reactions, including anaphylactic reactions, which can be fatal; Amoxil should not be given to penicillin-allergic patients.

What substances, supplements, or medications interact with Amoxicillin?

Amoxil may interact with sulfa medications, probenecid, blood thinners, and other antibiotics. Inform your doctor of every supplement and medication you take.

Amoxicillin Treatment During Pregnancy or Breastfeeding Should Be Used with Caution in Pregnant and Breastfeeding Women

Additional Information Our Amoxil Side Effects Drug Center offers a comprehensive overview of the drug information that is currently available regarding the potential effects that may occur while taking this medication.

Amoxicillin

An Overview Amoxicillin is an antibiotic

It is used to treat certain kinds of bacterial infections.

Amoxicillin oral tablets are available in chewable and immediate-release (IR) forms. Only generic medications are available for the chewable and IR tablets.

Amoxicillin is also available as a suspension and a capsule. All forms must be swallowed. This article centers around the oral tablet shapes as it were.)

Side effects of ampicillin The oral tablet of ampicillin does not make you sleepy, but it can have other side effects.

More typical adverse effects The most typical adverse effects of taking an oral amoxicillin tablet include:

Nausea, vomiting, diarrhea, a rash, and a vaginal yeast infection are all possible side effects that may pass in a few days or weeks. Talk to your pharmacist or doctor if they get worse or don't go away.

Serious side effects If you experience serious side effects, talk to your doctor right away. If you think you are experiencing a medical emergency or if your symptoms appear to be life-threatening, dial 911. The following are examples of serious side effects and how they can be felt:

Reactions to hypersensitivity. Some of the signs include:

a painful red or purple rash that spreads and leaves blisters that could cause the skin to break down and open sores, liver damage, or flu-like symptoms like a fever, body aches, or sore throat. Rarely does this happen. Some of the signs include:

a blood test shows an increase in liver enzymes, pain in the stomach, yellowing of the skin and eyes, fatigue, and a serious skin reaction. * This side effect rarely occurs. Some of the signs could be:

A skin rash and discoloration, swollen lymph nodes, itchiness, or other flu-like symptoms * Serious skin reactions were not reported in clinical trials of amoxicillin. However, since the drug's approval, they have been reported.

Disclaimer

Our objective is to offer you the most current and pertinent information. We cannot, however, guarantee that this information covers all possible side effects due to the fact that different people react differently to drugs. Do not rely solely on this information for medical advice. Always talk to a healthcare professional who knows your medical history about potential side effects.

Important warnings at the end of treatment

It's critical to follow your doctor's instructions and complete the amoxicillin treatment. If you start to feel better, don't stop taking this medication or skip doses. This may prolong the duration of your infection. It's also possible that you'll become resistant to the medication. As a result, you might not be able to use amoxicillin to treat a bacterial infection in the future.

Diarrhea: Diarrhea may be caused by amoxicillin. If you have bloody or watery diarrhea, fever, stomach cramps, or both, you should see a doctor.

Severe rashes on the skin: During treatment with amoxicillin, skin reactions may occur. Serious skin reactions like Steven-Johnson syndrome or toxic epidermal necrolysis can happen in very few cases. Converse with your primary care physician assuming you experience a skin rash or condition that becomes vexatious or doesn't disappear.

serious reaction to an allergen: This medication may trigger a severe allergic reaction. This reaction has the potential to result in death. Your risk of an allergic reaction may be higher if you are allergic to penicillins or cephalosporins, two types of antibiotics. While you are taking this medication, get in touch with your doctor right away if you experience breathing difficulties or tongue or throat swelling.

Amoxicillin: what is it?

Amoxicillin is an antibiotic that is prescribed. It is utilized to treat infections brought on by a particular strain of bacteria. It can be used in combination with other treatments. Because of this, you might have to take it with other medications.

There are two chewable and immediate-release (IR) forms of the oral tablet. Only generic drugs are available for these.

Nonexclusive medications as a rule cost less. Amoxicillin is also available as a suspension and a capsule. All structures are taken by mouth. The oral tablet forms are the sole focus of this article.

Amoxicillin is used because it is an antibiotic. It is utilized to treat infections brought on by a particular strain of bacteria.

Amoxicillin can be part of a treatment plan with other medications. Because of this, you might have to take it with other medications.

How it works: Amoxicillin is in the penicillin class of drugs. A class of medications is a gathering of meds that work likewise. These medications are much of the time used to treat comparative circumstances.

Amoxicillin stops bacteria from growing in your body and kills them.

How long it lasts Amoxicillin's effects should last as long as you keep taking it. Amoxicillin usually only works for a short time.

After your most recent dose, amoxicillin typically remains in your system for 8 to 12 hours. Even if you stop taking amoxicillin, you might continue to experience some of its side effects, especially during the 8- to 12-hour window. However, the drug usually stops working when your treatment is over or soon after.

People who stopped taking amoxicillin have been reported to have diarrhea that lasted for up to two months. Talk to your doctor if you stop taking amoxicillin and experience diarrhea along with a fever or abdominal pain.

After a dose, the oral amoxicillin tablets begin to work. The drug may not begin to reduce your infection's symptoms until several days after your first dose.

Talk to your doctor if you have any questions about the duration of amoxicillin treatment or its effects.

Cost of Amoxicillin

Like the prices of all medicines, amoxicillin can be expensive. The genuine cost you'll pay relies upon your protection plan, your area, and the drug store you use. For more information about how much treatment with amoxicillin costs, you can look at this article.

Assistance with money and insurance Some financial aid may be available to help you pay for amoxicillin.

Medicine Assistance Tool and NeedyMeds are two websites that provide resources for lowering the cost of amoxicillin. They also provide educational resources and tools to assist you in finding affordable healthcare. Go to their websites to find out more.

You can also save money on amoxicillin oral tablets by using the coupons in this article.

Check out this article to find out more about how to save money on prescription drugs.

Mail-order pharmacies A mail-order pharmacy might sell Amoxicillin. You might be able to get your medication without having to leave your house and save money by using this service.

Consult your physician, pharmacist, or insurance provider if you are interested in this option. Mail-order prescription drugs may be covered by some Medicare plans.

You can inquire about online pharmacy options from your doctor or pharmacist if you do not have insurance.

Amoxicillin dosage information for oral tablets is provided here. This may not cover all possible drug forms and dosages. The following factors will determine your drug's dosage, form, and frequency of use:

the severity of your condition, age, and any other medical conditions you may have, as well as how you responded to the first dose. Generic forms and strengths: Form of amoxicillin: oral tablet

Qualities: Form: 500 milligrams (875 mg) oral enjoyable tablet

Qualities: 250 mg and 125 mg Amoxicillin can also be taken orally in the form of a suspension or a capsule. The oral tablet forms are the sole focus of this article.

Adult dosage (age 18–64): IMMEDIATE-RELEASE TABLET AND CHEWABLE TABLET The usual dosage is 250 mg every 8 hours or 500 mg every 12 hours for infections of the ears, nose, and throat.

Dosage for children (ages 3 months to 17 years) is typically 25 mg per kilogram per day (mg/kg/day) divided into 12 equal doses and 20 mg/kg/day divided into 8 equal doses.

The dosage for children listed here is intended for children weighing less than 40 kilograms (88 pounds).

Dosing for children who weigh more than 88 pounds should follow adult recommendations.

Dosage for children (ages 0 to 2 months): The maximum daily dose is 30 mg/kg. Dosage information can be obtained from your child's doctor.

Adult dosage for urinary tract infections is 500 mg every 12 hours or 250 mg every 8 hours, depending on the patient's age.

Dosage for children (ages 3 months to 17 years) is typically 25 mg/kg/day divided into 12 equal doses or 20 mg/kg/day divided into 8 equal doses.

Dosage for children (ages 0 to 2 months): The maximum daily dose is 30 mg/kg. Dosage information can be obtained from your child's doctor.

Dosage for older adults (those 65 and older) The kidneys of older adults may not function as well as they once did. Your body may process drugs more slowly as a result of this. As a result, your body absorbs more of the drug over time. This makes you more likely to get side effects.

You might start on a lower dose or a different schedule for taking your medication. This can help prevent your body's levels of this drug from getting too high.

Special considerations regarding dosage for children: The dosage for children listed here is intended for children weighing less than 40 kilograms (88 pounds). Dosing for children who weigh more than 88 pounds should follow adult recommendations.

Adult dosage for skin infections is 500 mg every 12 hours or 250 mg every 8 hours, depending on the patient's age.

Dosage for children (ages 3 months to 17 years) is typically 25 mg/kg/day divided into 12 equal doses or 20 mg/kg/day divided into 8 equal doses.

This dosage is intended for children weighing less than 40 kilograms (88 pounds). Dosing for children who weigh more than 88 pounds should follow adult recommendations.

Dosage for children (ages 0 to 2 months): The maximum daily dose is 30 mg/kg. Dosage information can be obtained from your child's doctor.

Dosage for older adults (those 65 and older) The kidneys of older adults may not function as well as they once did. Your body may process drugs more slowly as a result of this. As a result, your body absorbs more of the drug over time. This makes you more likely to get side effects.

You might start on a lower dose or a different schedule for taking your medication. This can help prevent your body's levels of this drug from getting too high.

Adult dosage for lower respiratory tract infections is 875 mg every 12 hours or 500 mg every 8 hours, depending on the patient's age.

Dosage for children (ages 3 months to 17 years) is typically 40 mg/kg/day divided into 12 equal doses or 45 mg/kg/day divided into 8 equal doses.

Dosage for children (ages 0 to 2 months): The maximum daily dose is 30 mg/kg. This is intended for children under 40 kilograms (88 pounds). Dosing for children who weigh more than 88 pounds should follow adult recommendations. Dosage information can be obtained from your child's doctor.

Dosage for older adults (those 65 and older) The kidneys of older adults may not function as well as they once did. Your body may process drugs more slowly as a result of this. As a result, your body absorbs more of the drug over time. This makes you more likely to get side effects.

You might start on a lower dose or a different schedule for taking your medication. This can help prevent your body's levels of this drug from getting too high.

Gonorrhea dosage for adults (age 18–64): A single dose of 3 grams (g) is typical.

Dosage for children (24 months to 17 years): A single dose of 50 mg/kg of amoxicillin and 25 mg/kg of probenecid is common. The dosage for children listed here is intended for children weighing less than 40 kilograms (88 pounds).

Dosing for children who weigh more than 88 pounds should follow adult recommendations.

Dosage for children (ages 0 to 23 months): This medication should not be used to treat gonorrhea in children younger than 2 years old.

Dosage for older adults (those 65 and older) The kidneys of older adults may not function as well as they once did. Your body may process drugs more slowly as a result of this. As a result, your body absorbs more of the drug over time. This makes you more likely to get side effects.

You might start on a lower dose or a different schedule for taking your medication. This can help prevent your body's levels of this drug from getting too high.

Adult dosage (age 18–64) for stomach and intestinal ulcers The typical dosage for triple therapy is: For 14 days, 1 gram of amoxicillin, 500 mg of clarithromycin, and 30 mg of lansoprazole were administered twice daily.

Common doses for dual therapy include: For 14 days, 1 gram of amoxicillin and 30 milligrams of lansoprazole were taken three times daily.

Dosage for children (ages 0 to 17) This medication has not been studied for the treatment of stomach and intestinal ulcers in children.

Dosage for older adults (those 65 and older) The kidneys of older adults may not function as well as they once did. Your body may process drugs more slowly as a result of this. As a result, your body absorbs more of the drug over time. This makes you more likely to get side effects.

You might start on a lower dose or a different schedule for taking your medication. This can help prevent your body's levels of this drug from getting too high.

Disclaimer

Our objective is to offer you the most current and pertinent information. We cannot, however, guarantee that this list includes all possible dosages due to the fact that drugs affect different people in different ways. Do not rely solely on this information for medical advice. Always discuss the appropriate dosage with your doctor or pharmacist.

Amoxicillin oral tablet can interact with other medications, vitamins, or herbs that you may be taking. When a substance alters the way a drug works, this is called an interaction. This may be harmful or hinder the drug's effectiveness.

Your doctor should carefully manage all of your medications to help prevent interactions. Make sure to tell your doctor about any supplements, vitamins, or other medications you take.

Talk to your doctor or pharmacist about how this medication might interact with other medications you take.

The following is a list of drugs that may interact with amoxicillin.

Drugs that can make you more likely to get side effects from ampicillin Taking ampicillin with other drugs can make you more likely to get side effects from ampicillin. This is because there may be more amoxicillin in your body. Drugs like these are examples:

Probenecid: Amoxicillin levels in the blood could rise if probenecid is taken with it. Some patients might need less amoxicillin from their doctor.

Allopurinol: A rash may occur if you take amoxicillin and allopurinol at the same time.

Interactions with other drugs that make you more likely to get side effects When you take amoxicillin with other drugs, you are more likely to get side effects from those drugs. Amoxicillin makes your body have more of these drugs.

Blood thinners are one example of these medications. Anticoagulants (also known as blood thinners) include, among others, warfarin (Jantoven), apixaban (Eliquis), and heparin.

You run the risk of bleeding more often if you take these medications with amoxicillin. As a result, your doctor may alter your amoxicillin dosage.

When amoxicillin is less effective, interactions that can reduce its effectiveness Amoxicillin may not work as well when combined with certain medications. Studies conducted in vitro have demonstrated potential interactions that may result in a decrease in amoxicillin levels in the body.

Since in vitro examinations are just led in a lab and not on live subjects, it isn't evident whether this can essentially affect you on the off chance that you're taking amoxicillin with these medications.

Nevertheless, these drugs include the following:

Chloramphenicol If you take chloramphenicol and amoxicillin, your doctor probably won't change your dose.

Macrolides like erythromycin, clarithromycin, and azithromycin are examples of macrolides. If you take these medications together, your doctor probably won't change the amount of amoxicillin you take.

Sulfonamides like sulfamethoxazole: If you take these medications together, your doctor will probably give you the same amount of amoxicillin.

Tetracyclines, such as doxycycline or tetracycline, are examples of tetracyclines. If you take these medications together, your doctor might keep the same amount of amoxicillin for you.

When other drugs don't work as well: Amoxicillin and certain medications may not work as well together. This is because there may be less of these drugs in your body. Drugs like these are examples:

Oral contraceptives (also known as birth control) While taking amoxicillin, you should think about using a barrier method of birth control. Alternately, you might be given a different method of contraception by your doctor.

Disclaimer

Our objective is to offer you the most current and pertinent information. However, we cannot guarantee that this information covers all possible interactions because drug interactions vary from person to person. Do not rely solely on this information for medical advice. Make sure you talk to your doctor about any potential interactions you might have with any prescription, over-the-counter, or vitamins, herbs, or supplements you take.

Warns about Amoxicillin This medicine comes with a few warnings.

Allergic Reactions Amoxicillin can trigger severe allergic reactions. Some of the signs include:

difficulty breathing, swelling of the tongue or throat, or both If you experience an allergic reaction, contact your physician or America's Poison Centers at 800-222-1222 or through its online tool for assistance. Call 911 or go to the nearest ER if your symptoms are severe. If you have ever experienced an allergic reaction, do not take this medication again. Taking it again could be lethal (cause demise).

Precautions for individuals with specific medical conditions for individuals with mononucleosis (also known as kissing disease): Amoxicillin can make you more likely to get a severe rash.

for diabetic individuals: When testing for glucose (sugar) in the urine, amoxicillin may cause a false-positive reaction. While taking amoxicillin, talk to your doctor about how to control your blood sugar.

for kidney disease sufferers: It's possible that this medication won't be eliminated from your body as quickly if you have severe kidney disease. Amoxicillin levels may rise in your body as a result. Your physician may reduce your dosage of this medication to assist in preventing this.

Other groups that should be aware of: Pregnant women Amoxicillin exposure in pregnant animals has not been shown to have any negative effects on the fetus in animal studies. To determine whether the drug poses a threat to the fetus, insufficient human studies have been conducted. However, if you are pregnant or plan to become pregnant, you may still want to talk to your doctor.

Concerning those who are lactating (nursing): Amoxicillin might pass into bosom milk and may cause secondary effects in a youngster who is breastfed. If you are breastfeeding your child, talk to your doctor. You might have to decide whether to stop taking this medication or stop breastfeeding.

For individuals over the age of 65: It's possible that older people's kidneys aren't as effective as those of younger people. Your body may process drugs more slowly as a result of this. As a result, your body absorbs more of the drug over time. This makes you more likely to get side effects.

Amoxicillin oral tablets are taken as directed for short-term treatment. If you don't take it as directed, you run the risk of serious side effects.

If you suddenly stop taking the medication or don't take any at all: It's possible that your bacterial infection will not go away or get worse.

If you don't take the medication as directed or miss doses: It's possible that your medication won't work as well or won't work at all. A certain amount must always be present in your body for this medication to be effective.

It's critical to follow your doctor's treatment instructions to the letter. If you start to feel better, don't stop taking the medication or skip doses. This may prolong the duration of your infection.

It's also possible that you'll become resistant to the medication. This indicates that you may not be able to treat a bacterial infection with amoxicillin in the future.

If you consume in excess: You could have risky levels of the medication in your body. At less than 250 mg/kg, overdose symptoms may not be significant. It may cause kidney failure at higher doses.

If you think you've taken too much of this medication, call your doctor or use America's Poison Centers' online tool or call 800-222-1222. Call 911 right away or go to the nearest emergency room if your symptoms are severe.

If you miss a dose, what should you do?

As soon as you remember, take your medication. Take only one dose, however, if you remember just a few hours before your next scheduled dose. Do not attempt to catch up by taking two doses simultaneously. This could have harmful side effects.

How to determine whether the drug is working: Your infection's symptoms should subside.

Important things to keep in mind when taking amoxicillin Keep these things in mind if your doctor gives you an oral tablet of amoxicillin.

General: Take this medication according to your doctor's instructions.

The capsule, tablet, or suspension of amoxicillin can be taken with or without food.

Amoxicillin tablets can be broken up, cut, or chewed in any way you like.

Storage Keep amoxicillin at a temperature of 15 to 30 degrees Celsius at room temperature. Keep this drug out of direct sunlight. This medication should not be stored in bathrooms or other moist or damp areas.

Refills This medication's prescription may be refillable. This medication should be able to be refilled without requiring a new prescription. Your PCP will compose the quantity of reorders approved on your medicine.

Travel

While going with your drug:

Always keep your medications close by. Never put it in a checked bag while flying. It should be kept in your carry-on bag.

Don't worry about the X-ray machines at the airport. Your medication will not be harmed by them.

It's possible that you'll need to show the airport staff your medication's label. Keep the original prescription-labeled box with you at all times.

Do not leave this medication in your car or in the glove compartment. Make certain to try not to do this when the weather conditions are exceptionally sweltering or freezing.

Clinical monitoring You and your physician should keep an eye on specific health problems. This may assist in ensuring your safety while taking this medication. Your problems include:

Work of the kidneys. Your kidney function can be assessed through blood tests. Your doctor may decide to reduce your dose of this medication if your kidneys are not functioning properly.

Work of the liver. Your liver's efficiency can be determined by blood tests. Your doctor may reduce your dose of this medication if your liver is not functioning properly.

Your insurance company's coverage will determine how much these blood tests will cost.

Are there any other options?

You can treat your condition with other medications. Some might suit you better than others. Talk with your PCP about other medication choices that might work for you.

Disclaimer: Every effort has been made to ensure that all information in Medical News Today is accurate, complete, and current. However, a licensed healthcare professional's knowledge and experience should always take precedence over the information presented in this article. Before taking any medication, you should always talk to your doctor or another medical professional. This drug information is not meant to cover all possible uses, directions, precautions, warnings, drug interactions, allergic reactions, or adverse effects. It is subject to change. A drug or drug combination's absence of warnings or other information does not mean that it is safe, effective, or suitable for all patients or all uses.

Description: Amoxicillin, a semisynthetic antibiotic that is an analog of ampicillin and has broad bactericidal activity against numerous Gram-positive and Gram-negative microorganisms, is included in AMOXIL formulations. It is a chemical compound that is a trihydrate of (2S,5,R,6,R)-6-[(,R)-(-)-2-amino-2-(p-hydroxyphenyl)acetamido]-3,3-dimethyl-7-oxo-4-thia-1-azabicyclo[3.2.0]heptane-2-carboxylic acid.

Amoxicillin has a molecular weight of 419.45 and the formula $C_{16}H_{19}N_3O_5S \cdot 3H_2O$.

Capsules: The trihydrate of 250 mg or 500 mg of amoxicillin is contained in each AMOXIL capsule, which has a body that is opaque pink and a cap that is opaque royal blue. The product names AMOXIL and 250 are imprinted on both the capsule's body and cap; The letters AMOXIL and 500 are imprinted on both the capsule's body and cap. Ingredients that don't work: Red No. D&C 28, Blue FD&C No. 1, FD&C Red No. 40, titanium dioxide, magnesium stearate, and gelatin.

Tablets: Amoxicillin trihydrate, 500 mg or 875 mg, is present in each tablet. Each pink, film-coated, capsule-shaped tablet has AMOXIL centered over 500 or 875, respectively, debossed on it. On the back of the 875-mg tablet, there are scoring lines. Ingredients that don't work: FD&C Red No. 1, crospovidone, and colloidal silicon dioxide 30 percent aluminum lake, microcrystalline cellulose, hypromellose, magnesium stearate, polyethylene glycol, sodium starch glycolate, and titanium dioxide.

Oral Suspension Powder: Amoxicillin trihydrate amounts to 125 mg, 200 mg, 250 mg, or 400 mg in each 5 mL of reconstituted suspension. The 125-mg reconstituted suspension has 0.11 mEq (2.51 mg) of sodium in every 5 mL. The 200-mg reconstituted suspension has 0.15 mEq (3.39 mg) of sodium in every 5 mL. The 250-mg reconstituted suspension has 0.15 mEq (3.36 mg) of sodium in each 5 mL; The 400-mg reconstituted suspension has 0.19 mEq (4.33 mg) of sodium in each 5 mL container. Ingredients that don't work: Red FD&C No. 3, flavors, silicon dioxide, sodium bicarbonate, sodium citrate, sucrose, and xanthan gum

Indications Infections of the Ear, Nose, and Throat AMOXIL® is indicated for the treatment of infections caused by Streptococcus species that are susceptible (only -lactamase–negative) isolates. Streptococcus pneumoniae, Staphylococcus spp., and hemolytic isolates only or the influenza A virus.

Infections of The Genitourinary Tract

AMOXIL® can be used to treat infections caused by susceptible (ONLY -lactamase–negative) isolates of

Escherichia coli, Proteus mirabilis, or Enterococcus faecalis.

Skin and Skin Structure Infections AMOXIL® is used to treat infections caused by Streptococcus spp. that are susceptible (only -lactamase–negative) α-furthermore, β-hemolytic separates just), Staphylococcus spp., either E. coli

Lower Respiratory Tract Infections AMOXIL® is used to treat infections caused by Streptococcus spp. that are susceptible (only -lactamase–negative) Staphylococcus spp., S. pneumoniae, and hemolytic isolates only or H. pyogenes

Triple Therapy for Helicobacter Pylori with Clarithromycin and Lansoprazole is indicated for the treatment of patients with H. pylori infection and duodenal ulcer disease (active or 1-year history of a duodenal ulcer) to eradicate H. pylori. AMOXIL is used in conjunction with clarithromycin and lansoprazole. It has been demonstrated that eliminating H. pylori lowers the likelihood of duodenal ulcer recurrence.

Patients with H. pylori infection and duodenal ulcer disease (active or 1-year history of a duodenal ulcer) who are either allergic to clarithromycin or intolerant to it or in whom resistance to clarithromycin is known or suspected are eligible for dual therapy with lansoprazole AMOXIL and lansoprazole delayed-release capsules. Microbiology, the clarithromycin package insert.) It has been demonstrated that eliminating H. pylori lowers the likelihood of duodenal ulcer recurrence.

Use of AMOXIL (amoxicillin)

AMOXIL should only be used to treat infections that have been proven or strongly suspected to be caused by bacteria in order to maintain the effectiveness of AMOXIL (amoxicillin) and other antibacterial medications and prevent the development of drug-resistant bacteria. When selecting or modifying antibacterial therapy, culture and susceptibility information should be taken into consideration whenever they are available. Local epidemiology and susceptibility patterns may aid in the empiric selection of therapy in the absence of such data.

HOW SUPPLIED Dosage Forms and Strengths: 250 mg and 500 mg capsules The trihydrate of 250 mg or 500 mg of amoxicillin is contained in each AMOXIL capsule, which has a body that is opaque pink and a cap that is opaque royal blue. The product names AMOXIL and 250 are imprinted on both the capsule's body and cap; AMOXIL and 500 are imprinted on both the capsule's body and cap.

875 mg and 500 mg tablets. Amoxicillin trihydrate, 500 mg or 875 mg, is present in each tablet. Each film-covered, case molded, pink tablet is debossed with AMOXIL focused north of 500 or 875, individually. On the back of the 875-mg tablet, there are scoring lines.

Powder for Oral Suspension 125 mg/5 mL, 200 mg/5 mL, 250 mg/5 mL, and 400 mg/5 mL Each 5 mL of the strawberry-flavored trihydrate of the reconstituted suspension contains 125 mg of amoxicillin. Every 5 mL of reconstituted bubble-gumflavored suspension contains 200 mg, 250 mg or 400 mg amoxicillin as the trihydrate.

How to Handle and Store Capsules

The trihydrate of 250 mg or 500 mg of amoxicillin is contained in each AMOXIL capsule, which has a body that is opaque pink and a cap that is opaque royal blue. The product names AMOXIL and 250 are imprinted on both the capsule's body and cap; AMOXIL and 500 are imprinted on both the capsule's body and cap.

250-mg Container

NDC 43598-025-01 Jugs of 100

NDC 43598-025-05 Jugs of 500

500-mg Container

NDC 43598-005-01 Jugs of 100

NDC 43598-005-05 Jugs of 500

Tablets: Amoxicillin trihydrate, 500 mg or 875 mg, is present in each tablet. Each pink, film-coated, capsule-shaped tablet has AMOXIL centered over 500 or 875, respectively, debossed on it. On the back of the 875-mg tablet, there are scoring lines.

500-mg Tablet NDC 43598-024-01 100-mg Bottle NDC 43598-024-05 500-mg Bottle NDC 43598-019-

01 100-mg Bottle NDC 43598-019-14 20-mg Bottle Powder for Oral Suspension: Amoxicillin trihydrate is present in 125 mg per 5 milliliters of strawberry-flavored suspension that has been reconstituted. Amoxicillin trihydrate amounts to 200 mg, 250 mg, or 400 mg in each 5 mL of reconstituted bubble gum-flavored suspension.

200 mg/5 mL NDC 43598-023-50 50 mL NDC 43598-023-51 75 mL NDC 43598-023-52 100 mL NDC 43598-009-80 80 mL NDC 43598-009-52 100 mL NDC 43598-009-53 150 mL NDC 43598-007-50 50 mL NDC 43598-007-51 75 m

500 mg and 875 mg tablets, as well as 200 mg and 400 mg unreconstituted powder, should be kept at or below 25° C (77° F).

Use a tight container to distribute.

Precautions

Anaphylactic Reactions Patients receiving penicillin, including amoxicillin, have experienced severe and occasionally fatal hypersensitivity (anaphylactic) reactions. Anaphylaxis has occurred in patients taking oral penicillins, despite the fact that parenteral therapy is more common. People who have a history of penicillin hypersensitivity and/or sensitivity to multiple allergens are more likely to experience these reactions. There have been reports of people with a background marked by penicillin excessive touchiness who have encountered extreme responses when treated with cephalosporins. Prior to starting treatment with AMOXIL, cautious request ought to be made in regards to past extreme touchiness responses to penicillins, cephalosporins, or different allergens.

Diarrhea Caused by Clostridium Difficile Almost all antibacterial medications, including AMOXIL, have been linked to cases of CDAD, which can range in severity from mild diarrhea to fatal colitis. Antibacterial treatment alters the normal colonic flora, resulting in C. difficile overgrowth.

Toxins A and B produced by C. difficile aid in the development of CDAD. Due to the fact that these infections can be resistant to antimicrobial treatment and may necessitate colectomy, hypertoxin-producing strains of C. difficile result in increased morbidity and mortality. All patients who experience diarrhea following antibacterial treatment should be evaluated for CDAD. Since CDAD has been reported to occur more than two months after the administration of antibacterial agents, careful medical history is required.

Antibiotics that aren't meant for C. difficile may need to be stopped if CDAD is suspected or confirmed. When clinically necessary, appropriate fluid and electrolyte management, protein supplementation, C. difficile antibiotic treatment, and surgical evaluation should be implemented.

Use in Patients with Mononucleosis

A high percentage of patients with mononucleosis who receive amoxicillin develop an erythematous skin rash. Prescribing AMOXIL in the absence of a proven or strongly suspected bacterial infection is unlikely to benefit the patient and increases the risk of the development of drug-resistant bacteria. Patients with mononucleosis should not be given amoxicillin as a treatment.

Phenylketonurics The aspartame in the chewable Amoxil tablets contains phenylalanine. Phenylalanine is contained in 1.82 milligrams per 200 mg chewable tablet. Phenylalanine is present in 3.64 milligrams per 400 mg chewable tablet. Phenylketonurics can utilize the oral suspensions of Amoxil because they do not contain phenylalanine.

Nonclinical Toxicology Mutagenesis, Carcinogenesis, and Fertility Impairment There have not been any long-term studies in animals to evaluate the potential for carcinogenesis. There haven't been any studies done to see if amoxicillin alone can cause mutations; However, tests on a 4:1 mixture of amoxicillin and potassium clavulanate (AUGMENTIN) yield the following information. In both the yeast gene conversion assay and the Ames bacterial mutation assay, AUGMENTIN did not cause mutations. In the mouse lymphoma assay, AUGMENTIN was only slightly positive, but the assay's trend toward increased mutation frequencies occurred at doses that were also associated with decreased cell survival. In both the mouse dominant lethal assay and the mouse micronucleus test, AUGMENTIN failed. In both the mouse micronucleus test and the Ames bacterial mutation assay, potassium clavulanate alone failed all of the tests. At doses up to 500 mg/kg (approximately two times the human dose of 3 g based on body surface area), rats in a multigenerational reproduction study showed no impairment of fertility or other adverse reproductive effects.

Use in Specific Populations Pregnancy Teratogenic Effects Pregnancy Category B. Mice and rats have been used in reproduction studies at doses up to 2000 mg/kg, which is three and six times the human dose of three grams, depending on body surface area. Amoxicillin did not appear to harm the fetus in any way. However, no adequate and well-controlled studies have been conducted on pregnant women. Amoxicillin should only be used during pregnancy if absolutely necessary due to the fact that studies on animal reproduction are not always able to predict how humans will react.

During Pregnancy and Childbirth Oral ampicillin is poorly absorbed. Amoxicillin use in humans during labor or delivery is not known to have any effect on the fetus immediately or later, prolong labor, or increase the likelihood of an obstetrical intervention being required.

Penicillins have been shown to be excreted in human milk by nursing mothers. The use of amoxicillin by pregnant women may make their infants more sensitive. When administering amoxicillin to a woman who is nursing, extreme caution should be taken.

Amoxicillin's elimination may be delayed in infants and young children due to their incomplete renal development. Pediatric patients younger than 12 weeks (less than 3 months) should have their AMOXIL doses adjusted.

Geriatric Use

An examination of clinical investigations of AMOXIL was directed to decide if subjects matured 65 and over answer uniquely in contrast to more youthful subjects. Although there are no differences in responses between older and younger patients, it is possible that some older people are more sensitive.

Since the kidney is known to excrete a significant amount of this medication, patients with impaired renal function may be more likely to experience toxic reactions. Dosage selection and monitoring of renal function should be carefully considered because elderly patients are more likely to have impaired renal function.

Dosing in Patients with Renal Impairment Because amoxicillin is primarily eliminated by the kidney, patients with severe renal impairment (GFR 30 mL/min) typically require dosage adjustments. For specific recommendations for patients with renal impairment, see Dosing in Renal Impairment.

Overdosage and Contraindications

OVERDOSE in the event of an overdose, stop taking the medication, treat the symptoms, and take any necessary supportive measures. A prospective study of 51 children at a poison control center found that amoxicillin overdoses of less than 250 mg/kg did not cause significant clinical symptoms.

Overdosage of amoxicillin has been associated with a small number of cases of interstitial nephritis and oliguric renal failure.

Amoxicillin overdose in both adult and pediatric patients has also been associated with crystalluria, which can sometimes result in renal failure. In the event of an overdose, diuresis and adequate fluid intake should be maintained to lower the risk of amoxicillin crystalluria.

Drug administration cessation appears to reverse renal impairment. Due to decreased renal clearance of amoxicillin, patients with impaired renal function may experience higher blood levels more frequently. Hemodialysis can remove amoxicillin from the bloodstream.

CONTRAINDICATIONS Patients who have had a severe hypersensitivity reaction (such as anaphylaxis or Stevens-Johnson syndrome) to AMOXIL or to other

-lactam antibiotics (such as penicillins and cephalosporins) are not advised to take AMOXIL.

Mechanism of Action in Clinical Pharmacology
Amoxicillin is an antibacterial drug.

Pharmacokinetics Absorption Amoxicillin is rapidly absorbed when taken orally and remains stable in the presence of gastric acid. A portion of an investigation has looked into how food affects how amoxicillin from tablets and suspension is absorbed; The 400-mg and 875-mg formulations have only been studied when taken before a light meal.

Average peak blood levels of 250-mg and 500-mg amoxicillin capsules administered orally range from 3.5 to 5.0 mcg/mL and 5.5 to 7.5 mcg/mL, respectively, 1 to 2 hours after administration.

An open, two-part, single-dose crossover bioequivalence study comparing 875 mg of AMOXIL to 875 mg of AUGMENTIN® (amoxicillin/clavulanate potassium) in 27 adults revealed that the 875 mg tablet of AMOXIL produces an AUC_0- of 35.4 8.1

mcg•hr/mL and a Cmax of 13.8 4.1 mcg/mL at the beginning of a light

Orally directed portions of amoxicillin suspension, 125 mg/5 mL and 250 mg/5 mL, bring about normal pinnacle blood levels 1 to 2 hours after organization in the scope of 1.5 mcg/mL to 3.0 mcg/mL and 3.5 mcg/mL to 5.0 mcg/mL, separately.

The majority of the body's tissues and fluids are easily absorbed by ampicillin, with the exception of the brain and spinal fluid when meninges are inflamed. Amoxicillin is about 20% protein-bound in blood serum. Therapeutic levels of the antibiotic were found in the interstitial fluid following a one-gram dose and a special skin window method for determining levels.

Amoxicillin has a half-life of 61.3 minutes in metabolism and elimination. Within six to eight hours, approximately sixty percent of an oral dose of amoxicillin is excreted in the urine. Amoxicillin can be taken orally, and up to eight hours later, serum levels that can be detected are observed. Concurrent administration of probenecid can delay the excretion of amoxicillin because most of it is excreted unchanged in the urine.

Microbiology Mechanism of Action Amoxicillin's bactericidal effect on susceptible bacteria during active multiplication is comparable to that of penicillin. The bacteria die as a result of its action, which prevents the biosynthesis of the cell wall.

Amoxicillin resistance is primarily caused by enzymes known as beta-lactamases that cleave the beta-lactam ring of the antibiotic, rendering it inactive.

According to the INDICATIONS AND USAGE section, amoxicillin has been shown to be effective against the majority of the bacterial isolates listed below, both in clinical infections and in vitro.

Gram-Positive Bacteria Staphylococcus Spp. Enterococcus faecalis

Streptococcus pneumoniae and other species Gram-Negative Bacteria (alpha and beta-hemolytic) Escherichia coli Haemophilus influenzae Helicobacter pylori Proteus mirabilis Susceptibility Test Methods When available, the clinical microbiology laboratory should provide the physician with periodic reports that describe the susceptibility profile of nosocomial and community-acquired pathogens. These reports should include cumulative in vitro susceptibility test results for antimicrobial drugs The doctor should be able to use these reports to choose the best antimicrobial.

Techniques for Diluting: The minimum inhibitory concentrations (MICs) of antimicrobials are determined using quantitative techniques. Estimates of bacteria's susceptibility to antimicrobial compounds are provided by these MICs. A standardized test (broth or agar) should be used to determine the MICs2,4. The criteria in Table 4 should be used to interpret the MIC values.

Techniques for Diffusion: Additionally, reproducible estimates of the susceptibility of bacteria to antimicrobial compounds can be provided by quantitative methods that require the measurement of zone diameters3,4. A standard test strategy should be used to determine the size of the zone3.

Amoxicillin-resistant Enterococcus species, by testing ampicillin4, enterobacteriaceae and H. influenzae can be inferred. Staphylococcus spp. amoxicillin sensitivity, and Streptococcus spp. beta-hemolytic, could be deduced from testing penicillin4. The majority of Enterococcus spp. isolates that produce a beta-lactamase of the TEM type and are resistant to ampicillin or amoxicillin. A quick method for determining resistance to ampicillin and amoxicillin4 is a beta-lactamase test.

Penicillin or oxacillin testing can be used to determine whether non-meningitis Streptococcus pneumoniae isolates are susceptible to amoxicillin.

If the antimicrobial compound reaches a concentration at the infection site necessary to inhibit pathogen growth, a report of "Susceptible" indicates that the antimicrobial is likely to do so. A report of "Intermediate" means that the result should be considered ambiguous and that the test should be repeated if the microorganism is not fully susceptible to alternative, clinically feasible drugs. This category indicates that the drug may have clinical application in physiologically concentrated areas of the body. In addition, this category serves as a buffer zone, preventing minor, uncontrollable technical factors from leading to significant interpretational inconsistencies. If the antimicrobial compound reaches the concentration typically achievable at the infection site, a report of "Resistant" indicates that it is unlikely to inhibit pathogen growth. A different treatment should be chosen.

Amoxicillin in vitro susceptibility testing methods for determining minimum inhibitory concentrations (MICs) and zone sizes for the testing of Helicobacter pylori have not been standardized, validated, or approved. Patients who fail triple therapy should have specimens tested for H. pylori and clarithromycin susceptibility tested. A regimen that does not contain clarithromycin ought to be used if resistance to clarithromycin is discovered.

Quality Control Standardized susceptibility test procedures[2,3,4] necessitate the use of laboratory controls to monitor and guarantee the precision of the supplies and reagents used in the assay, as well as the methods employed by those carrying out the test control.

Medication Guide PATIENT INFORMATION Patients should be informed that, depending on the prescribed dose, AMOXIL can be taken every 8 hours or every 12 hours.

It is important to inform patients that antibiotics, such as AMOXIL, should only be used to treat bacterial infections. They do not treat viruses like the common cold. Patients who receive a prescription for AMOXIL to treat a bacterial infection should be informed that, despite the fact that it is common for patients to feel better early on in the treatment, the medication should be taken exactly as prescribed. If you miss a dose or don't finish the treatment, it can: 1) make the immediate treatment less effective, and 2) make it more likely that bacteria will develop resistance and become untreatable with AMOXIL or other antibacterial medications in the future.

It is important to inform patients that antibiotic-caused diarrhea typically subsides when the medication is stopped. Patients may experience bloody and watery stools (with or without fever and stomach cramps) after beginning antibiotic treatment, even two or more months after receiving their last dose. Patients should get in touch with their doctor as soon as possible if this happens.

AMOXIL contains a drug product of the penicillin class, which may cause allergic reactions in some patients.

EARS INJURIES IN CHILDREN AND ADULTS

At times, it may appear as though kids always get ear infections. Children are very likely to get ear infections. About twice as often as they get a cold, children get ear infections. Because children's small ears don't drain fluid as well as adults' do, they are more likely to get ear infections. Additionally, children's immune systems are still developing, which makes certain infections more likely.

Ear infections come in three varieties. The location in the ear canal where they occur defines each type. The inner, middle, or outer ear are all possible locations for an ear infection. The symptoms of each kind of ear infection may vary.

SWIMMER'S EAR (OUTER EAR INFECTION)

Swimmer's ear refers to an infection of the ear canal, also known as the outer ear. The fact that the ear canal stays wet long enough for bacteria or other organisms to grow is what gives it its name.

Swimmer's ear is caused by bacteria and fungi, and the skin that covers the ear canal and outer ear protects against them. However, bacteria or fungi can enter the ear and cause infection if this skin barrier is breached. An outer ear infection or swimmer's ear is the name given to this ear infection. Either putting something too deeply into the ear or having too much moisture in the ear canal can cause swimmer's ear.

The acidic environment of the ear canal is altered when swimming or showering, allowing bacteria or fungi to enter the ear. When cotton swabs or other objects are inserted into the ear, they can also scratch or injure the lining of the ear canal, breaking it. Chemicals that irritate the ear canal and skin conditions that cause the skin to crack are additional causes of swimmer's ear.

Symptoms of Swimmer's

Ear Swimmer's ear typically causes pain. Over the course of a few days, swimmer's ear pain gradually begins. When the ear is touched, pulled, or chewed, the pain is especially bad. The following are swimmer's ear symptoms:

Fluid crusting at the opening of the ear canal Trouble Hearing Ringing in the ear (tinnitus) and dizziness or spinning sensation (vertigo) Feeling of fullness in the ear Pain on the side of the face or neck Swollen lymph nodes Swimmer's Ear Treatment: Drops and Home Remedies: Swimmer's ear treatment options include not swimming, taking over-the-counter painkillers, and possibly antibiotics. Medication that relieves symptoms and cleans the affected ear may be prescribed by doctors. Application of heat to the ear with a heating pad and a rinse with white vinegar to help restore the ear canal's natural pH and reduce swelling are home remedies for swimmer's ear.

EAR INFECTION DIAGNOSIS

Using an otoscope, the inside of the ear is examined to determine the presence of an infection. The color shown here is pinkish-gray in an eardrum that is healthy and normal. An infected eardrum is reddened and bulging, whereas a healthy eardrum is clear. Tympanometry, which measures how the eardrum responds to a change in air pressure inside the ear, can also be done by a doctor. When a child has fluid in both ears, hearing tests are another common way to diagnose an ear infection. If there are indications of immune issues, blood tests may also be performed.

INFECTION OF THE MIDDLE EARS

Bacteria and viruses are the main culprits in middle ear infections. An allergy or upper respiratory infection can cause swelling that can obstruct the Eustachian tubes, preventing air from reaching the middle ear. After that, germs and fluid are pulled into the middle ear by a vacuum and suction. The fluid can't flow out of the tubes because they are swollen. A medium for the growth of viruses or bacteria that cause middle ear infections is provided by this.

To determine whether the eardrum vibrates normally, the otoscope can blow a small amount of air against it. The eardrum does not normally vibrate when there is fluid in the middle ear.

Eustachian Tube The canal that runs from your middle ear to your throat is called the Eustachian tube. The Eustachian tube keeps air and fluid pressure from building up inside the ear when it is open as it should be. The Eustachian tube can become swollen and blocked by infections like the common cold, the flu, or allergic reactions.

Middle Ear Infection Symptoms

Middle ear infections typically present themselves between two and seven days after the onset of a cold or other respiratory infection. Symptoms of a middle ear infection include:

Ear pain that ranges from mild to severe Fever Drainage from the ear that is thick, yellow, or bloody

Appetite loss, vomiting, and grumpy behavior Trouble sleeping Middle Ear Infection Treatment The majority of the time, the treatment for middle ear infections focuses on reducing pain. Acetaminophen and ibuprofen, two common over-the-counter medications for fever and pain, are used. Importantly, never give children aspirin. Despite the fact that antibiotics may be prescribed for middle ear infections, they typically improve on their own. A doctor might prescribe oral antibiotics for a long time to children who keep getting ear infections. Children who experience recurrent middle ear infections may also benefit from having ear tubes inserted or their tonsils or adenoids removed.

INFLECTION OF THE INSIDE OF THE EARS (LABYRINTHITIS)

Labyrinthitis is an inflammation of the inner ear. When the labyrinth, a part of the inner ear that helps you stay balanced, gets swollen, you get labyrinthitis. Ear infections, both viral and bacterial, and respiratory illnesses can all contribute to the labyrinth's inflammation.

Symptoms of an Inner Ear Infection

The signs and symptoms of an inner ear infection can be quite intense for several days. The signs and symptoms of an inner ear infection include:

Vertigo (dizziness with the sensation of moving), tinnitus (ringing or buzzing in the ear), and difficulty focusing the eyes are all symptoms of inner ear infection. Treatment for inner ear infection typically entails taking sedatives, corticosteroids, and prescription and over-the-counter antihistamines to manage symptoms. If there is an active infection, antibiotics might be prescribed. Treatments for vertigo include the following:

The eardrum can rupture when the pressure from fluid buildup is too high inside the middle ear, as shown here. Sit still during a vertigo attack. Get up slowly if lying down or seated. Avoid bright screens or flashing lights during a vertigo attack. Use low light rather than darkness or bright lights. Fluid that is brown, yellow, or white can drain from the ear when the eardrum bursts. When the eardrum bursts, the pressure is released, and the pain may suddenly subside.

Symptoms of a Ruptured Eardrum

A ruptured eardrum can present with numerous symptoms. However, the sound of air blowing out of the ear when you blow your nose and an uncomfortable feeling in the ear are the most common signs of a ruptured eardrum. Another symptom of a ruptured eardrum is as follows:

Ruptured Eardrum Treatment

The eardrum typically heals without medical treatment within a few weeks after a rupture, and hearing is typically not worsened unless rupture and/or infection continues to occur frequently over a period of time. Sudden sharp ear pain or a sudden decrease in ear pain Drainage from the ear that may be bloody, clear, or resemble pus Ear noise or buzzing Hearing loss that may be partial or complete in the affected ear Episodic Ear Anti-microbials might be recommended to forestall an ear contamination. If the ruptured eardrum is causing pain, prescription painkillers may also be recommended. The rupture may necessitate surgery to repair the eardrum. A piece of your own tissue, typically from above the ear, will be attached to the eardrum for reconstruction if this is the case.

SYMPTOMS OF EAR INFECTION

In children, ear pain is the most common symptom of an ear infection. Due to the pain, children who have ear infections may have difficulty sleeping. Other symptoms include ear discharge or fluid, fever, hearing issues, dizziness, and congestion in the nose. The signs of fluid buildup include:

A feeling of fullness or pressure in the ear, popping, ringing, or trouble hearing Children may rub their ears to relieve pressure. Children who have trouble hearing may appear dreamy or unfocused, as well as irritable or grumpy. Balance issues and dizziness

www.ingramcontent.com/pod-product-compliance
Lightning Source LLC
Chambersburg PA
CBHW070130230526
45472CB00004B/1495